I0440036

First Light of Dawn

L.S. Elmer

Copyright © 2012 L.S. Elmer

All rights reserved.

ISBN -10:148115656X

ISBN-13: 978 - 1481156561

DEDICATION

So this is the bit where I am supposed to be nice to
people. Where I am supposed to thank everyone for their
ongoing support and for all the help I have received in
creating this book. Totally unoriginal! So I'm going to say
what I want to say instead.........

To all my friends and family – you drive me absolutely
crazy......... but I love you all to bits! Thanks for letting
me drive you crazy too.

CONTENTS

ACKNOWLEDGMENTS

Copyright © L.S.Elmer 2012

The right of Linda Elmer to be identified as the author of this
work has been asserted by her in accordance with the
Copyright, Design and Patents Act 1988
Cover design and layout by L.S. Elmer

Please seek advice from your doctor before undertaking any
changes to your daily routine to ensure that you are receiving
the best care possible.

All characters in this book are fictitious and any resemblance to
actual persons, living or dead, is purely coincidental.
All rights reserved. No part of this publication may be reproduced,
stored in a retrieval system, or transmitted, in any form or by any
means, electronic, mechanical, photocopying, recording or otherwise,
without the prior permission of the publishers.
This book is sold subject to the condition that it shall not, by way of
trade or otherwise, be lent, re-sold, hired out or otherwise circulated
without the publisher's prior consent in any form of binding or cover
other than that in which it is published and without a similar condition
including this condition being imposed on the subsequent purchaser.

1 INTRODUCTION

When most people start out on their M.E. journey they find themselves surrounded by a mist of confusion. This has nothing to do with the fact that the condition causes you to feel like this, it is just that there are so many mysteries surrounding it, that it is hard to work out what is going on.

We read books, listen to advice, do exactly what our GP tells us. And all of this adds up to not feeling better and not knowing when we will. Not very helpful I hear you say. All of the advice out there tells us that there are no answers. So we listen to everything and anything that might provide a cure; but nine times out of ten........it doesn't.

In my own experience of the condition I found myself questioning the advice I was given. There was some logic to it: but the more I asked questions, the more I found out that the answers were staring me right in the face. They were already there but they just needed a bit of changing in order for me to get better.

Once I finally realized a few things I slowly went from strength to strength. The progress was slow and steady so I didn't realize it straight away. But the techniques I used led me from severe M.E. to total recovery.

I am not going to promise any miracle cures in this book. I don't have any. But what I can say is that the answers I have discovered have enabled me to find solutions to what has previously been shrouded in mystery.

2 HOW THE BRAIN WORKS

What causes M.E.?

If you are expecting some extremely scientific theory at this point you will be very disappointed. Everything I can tell you is based on a lot of research done by others, and the combining of everything that they have found out. When you put it all together though, common sense will tell you everything that you need to know about the condition.

To understand what is happening with M.E. it is necessary to look at all of the different factors involved. First, let's look at the things known to cause the illness.

The following are a list of things that patients commonly

report as having triggered the onset of their illness. In some cases people do not know the cause, but this list tends to be the main things quoted.

- Viral Infection
- Immunisation
- Traumatic or Stressful Event
- Childhood Abuse

When put together, these things at first seem completely unconnected, but when you look a bit further there is actually a clear link between them. They all create additional hormones in the body that are not generally present in day to day circumstances.

Why is the Hypothalamus so Important?

Let's look at the original triggers of M.E., all of them have a potential link to the hypothalamus.

1. Viral Infection – In a viral infection the body tries to fight off the infection through the immune system. Without going in to too much detail, the hypothalamus is the thing that controls the immune system. It has to work really hard when we are unwell to try to do this. If it has previous experience of a particular illness then it is able to

4

do this more easily but when it is fighting something new it can be a lot harder.

2. Immunisation – Immunisation works by introducing a small amount of an illness into your body so that your body learns how to fight it off. It is better able to defend itself if it comes across the real thing later on. This is again controlled by the hypothalamus.

3. Traumatic or Stressful Events – When exposed to traumatic or stressful events, the body prepares itself to either fight or run away. It does this by increasing hormones such as adrenaline. Our bodies are designed to cope with this in the wild if we were for example being attacked by a lion. We would temporarily be prepared to defend ourselves but this would quickly either be successful or unsuccessful. We are designed to be able to cope with such stress for only a short period of time. If left feeling like this for a long period of time the hormones produced by the hypothalamus can have a very negative effect on the body.

4. Childhood Abuse – Just as with any other stressful situation, the body prepares to defend itself. In this case however, it is exposed to high levels of stress hormones for a long period of time, which the body is not designed to cope with.

It may be that you experienced either one or more of these situations at the time of onset of your illness. Regardless of what happened, the evidence suggests that in all cases, the hypothalamus was put under a lot of pressure. Why this leads to some people developing M.E. and not others I cannot say. But if the hypothalamus has become overwhelmed then it should only need the opportunity to reprogram itself in order for the patient to make a full recovery. As with any illness, the body's best chance to heal itself is when it is allowed to rest.

What do the symptoms tell us?

Scientists have often tried to separate the condition into different illnesses, as the onset circumstances are often different from one patient to the next. This has led to M.E. being called various different things such as Post-Viral Fatigue, Chronic Fatigue Syndrome etc., but the fact remains that they all produce a very similar set of symptoms regardless of what originally caused the patient to be unwell.

If you look at appendix 1, you will find a full list of symptoms that M.E. patients tend to experience. This is a very thorough list so please be aware that some of these symptoms are only experienced by patients in the very severe stage of the condition.

All of the symptoms on this list are in some way connected to the hypothalamus. The hypothalamus controls most of the body's functions by introducing hormones that tell the body what to do and when. As every symptom is connected to this part of the brain this is yet more evidence that the hypothalamus is the key factor in M.E.

M.E. patients tend to find that the more exhausted they are and the worse their condition, the more symptoms they experience. As they feel better the symptoms are lessened, and if this continues then they find that the symptoms gradually disappear.

A lot of people tend to find that although they rest, their condition seems to fluctuate at random. This is not actually the case. When most people think of resting, they think of resting the body. They think of lying down, sleeping, not going out or doing much. This is all very well when it comes to allowing the body to rest but it does very little for the hypothalamus.

What treatments work and what happens when patients are not able to heal?

More evidence that the hypothalamus is key to the condition can be found when we look at the current treatments that are known to successfully help M.E. patients. By looking at these individually we can clearly see that they all suggest that allowing the hypothalamus to rest is the best course of action in treating M.E.

- Anti-depressant medication
- Resting
- Any medication that treats their current symptoms
- Stress reduction techniques

Each of these treatments that have had some success have allowed something connected to the hypothalamus to rest. For example, lowering stress, allowing the body to rest, supporting the body's symptoms so that the hypothalamus does not have to work as hard, all apply to the points previously mentioned. It follows that if we work on all areas of the hypothalamus that can be rested at the same time that most patients are likely to make significant progress towards a full recovery.

Let's also look at cases where patients have been unable to make any real progress for a significant length of time. This is a list of things that tend to apply in these cases. If this situation applies to you then look at this list and see how many of these things are relevant in your case.

- Have been left undiagnosed for a long period of time.

- Do not have much support from family and friends
- Do not have a lot of support from their GP/Specialist.
- Have continued to do normal activities such as studying or working despite feeling ill.
- Have participated in activity management programs where they are encouraged to continue a level of activity appropriate to them at all times.
- Have trouble maintaining their finances due to their condition.
- Have become isolated.
- Have developed depression as a result of their situation.
- Have given up believing that they can recover

I will make an educated guess on this one. If several of these things apply to you then you are probably finding that your condition is getting worse or you are already in the severe stage of it. Am I right? If so,.....keep reading.

For those who originally experienced either trauma or childhood abuse at the onset of their illness it is important to check that they are no longer experiencing these situations if they are going to be able to recover. Even after the event itself, it is possible that flashbacks and nightmares of the event can lead to ongoing stress that may prevent the patient from recovering. If this may be the case then support needs to be provided for this separately.

How can we give the Hypothalamus chance to heal?

This is all good in theory but how does it work in practice. If the hypothalamus is malfunctioning due to being overwhelmed then the best way to let it heal is to not allow it to be any further stimulated than necessary. This probably sounds a little complicated to achieve but in practice there are a few clear steps that should allow you to do this.

- Eliminate as much stress as possible so that the amount of hormones introduced into the body can be reduced.
- Use medication to treat severe symptoms.
- Avoid further illnesses such as flu or colds.
- Allow both the body and mind as much time to rest as they need.
- Do not allow yourself to become mentally over stimulated. The hypothalamus controls how the brain processes information so giving it a limited amount to work on will help.

In reading the following chapters you should come to a clear understanding of what you need to do to be able to achieve this.

Remember……it is the hypothalamus that needs to rest and not just the body.

Scientists have not currently determined what the cause of M.E. is but any of them will tell you that the brain is an extremely complicated thing and there is so much that we don't know about it. It may take many years for a full answer to be given but that doesn't mean that we can't find the answers that we need.

3 STRESS

<u>How stress affects the body</u>

The first thing any patient with M.E. thinks when they hear about the link between stress and the worsening of the condition, is that this is yet another attempt at people convincing you that the illness is psychological. But it isn't. Studies have shown a clear link between M.E. becoming worse when someone is regularly stressed, as well as it taking longer for a person to recover. So what is the reason for this?

When stressed the body produces a range of hormones that have a very negative effect on the body. This has been shown to be the case in many people who do not have M.E., so it is hardly surprising that it has a very bad effect in patients whose bodies react badly to anything that will cause the hypothalamus to work harder than normal.

While there are many hormonal factors at play in M.E, the worst thing possible is the introduction of stress related hormones. It is therefore vital that these are eliminated as much as possible if a patient is going to be able to make steady progress towards getting well. Stress is in fact probably the biggest reason why M.E. patients are unable to recover effectively, and the following sections will help to highlight why this is such an important factor.

It has long been recognised that young people with M.E. tend to make a quicker recovery than adults. While this may be due to their bodies being younger and more able to heal themselves, there is also another big factor that is likely to be playing a part. Those under 18 do not tend to have finances to worry about, they do not need to worry about their career as this can be picked up later on, they tend to have a lot more support from their families, they generally get less accusations from people about faking it......and the list goes on. It is easier also at this age to be able to take a gap year from their studies which again is extremely helpful towards making a full recovery.

The important thing to remember

The worst cause of stress for M.E. patients is that they

have no idea when they are going to get better, how long it will take or if it will even happen. They eventually give up on the idea of ever being well again and lose all faith that miracles can happen. Of course what happens then is that they spiral into depression, feel extremely stressed and the M.E. gets a lot worse.

If you are going to get better you have to believe that you will. There is nothing more important in your recovery than this. Know it will happen. Plan for when it will. This is the best medicine that anyone can ever give you.

I can tell you from experience that after living with M.E. for fifteen years I too felt like it would never end.........but it did!

Managing your finances

It goes without saying that the highest priority for any M.E. patient is to focus on organising their finances. Even if you are unable to do anything else this must be dealt with first. There is nothing more stressful than knowing that you are too ill to go out to work and worrying about whether you have enough money to feed yourself or to keep your home.

Use any time that you are feeling well to arrange your finances so that you do not have to worry about this later on. There are many agencies out there who can support you with this and if you explain that you struggle to complete the forms due to your condition, further support can be provided. The main people to contact in the UK are:

- Citizen's Advice Bureau
- Job Centre
- Local Council

The first two agencies can help you with claiming Disability Living Allowance (DLA) and Employment and Support Allowance (ESA). The council will help you with claiming Housing Benefit which you will be entitled to if you are on a low income. They may also help you to address your housing needs if your current accommodation isn't suitable. Social Services could also provide further support, particularly if your condition is severe and you do not have a relative who can act as a carer.

Agencies such as these tend to put very specific deadlines on their applications. If you are unable to meet these due to ill health however, make sure that you phone them as they will probably extend this if required, so long as you keep in contact with them so that they know what is happening.

Dealing with personal relationships

It is very important that those close to you are as aware of your condition as possible due to the numerous misconceptions that are commonly held. A lack of knowledge and understanding can often lead to breakdown in relationships that could otherwise have been prevented. It is needless to say that strain between friends and family is another common source of stress for M.E. patients but this is also an area that can be worked on if this is carefully addressed. In the past, a lack of support in society and negative views portrayed by the media, have often influenced the views of family and friends. But thankfully this is beginning to change. More and more people are able to get the support that they need simply because of better information and more people being aware that this is a serious condition that has a very negative affect on peoples' lives. Please refer to Chapter 6 for further advice on this matter.

Fatigue can often make it hard to speak in social settings as this uses up energy. It is often the case though that a patient can benefit from being around others talking, even though they are unable to participate fully in the conversation themselves. It is easy for people to think that they do not want to join in as they do not say much when there, but just being around normal life and listening to everyday conversation can be very beneficial.

Being Yourself

Many of us who have M.E. previously led very active or possibly intellectual lives that we are now not able to do. The condition prevents us from doing a lot of things and some of these things are an important part of who we are as individuals. This can make you feel like you are no longer yourself and this is beyond frustrating. For this reason, knowing that you will get better is a very important factor.

If you know that you will get better then it is simply a matter of time before you can be yourself again. This being the case, there is no harm in surrounding yourself with the things that remind you of who you really are. It is really important to do this. Some days we can end up feeling so ill that we feel as if we are an illness and not a human being. This is dangerous thinking. If you are an artist then put up paintings. Don't hide them because you are not able to paint at the moment. If you used to be active then fill your room with all the things that you used to use on a regular basis. Put up pictures of the days when you felt most like yourself. Some people say that this is not recognising that you are now ill and call it denial….personally I call it self-acceptance and belief. Know that one day you will be able to do those things again and try not to be too frustrated because you can't do them temporarily.

De-stressing tips for when you can't do much

Having M.E. can understandably lead to depression which is a normal response to the situation you find yourself in. As this will have a negative effect on your body due to the hormones produced through feeling depressed, it is important to treat this as soon as possible. Failure to do so is likely to bring on more problems with your M.E. such as frequent relapses and a general worsening of your condition.

If stress is properly managed however, the risk of this happening can be kept to an absolute minimum which gives the patient a strong chance to recover.

It is very important that every day, regardless of how ill you feel, that you take some time to enjoy yourself and de-stress. Please refer to appendix 2: Daily Diary and use this to remind yourself of the importance of making this a daily priority.

If you do nothing but focus on de-stressing in your quest to get better, you will still make significant improvement towards getting well.

The list below contains some suggestions of things you can do while ill. See how many more you can think of that would be good for you. You may be surprised at how many simple things you can actually find.

Warning! Some of these suggestions are extremely childish so anyone who doesn't like that sort of thing had better not read this list.

Falling asleep in the strangest of places

Having a cup of tea in the garden, listening to the birds sing and feeling the sunshine warm your body

Putting candles around the edge of the bath and enjoying a nice scented bubble bath.

Saying hello to a pet cat that has wandered into your garden.

Watching a fast paced action film and imagining you're actually driving the car yourself.

Watching a program on TV about blowing stuff up –
children's science programs are always good for that.

Watching a comedy (don't watch any sad films until
you feel better)!

Keeping in touch with people via email or the internet.

Painting

Gardening while sat down

Growing a sunflower from seed, you can watch it
grow even if you are in bed and those plants won't
allow anyone to feel miserable.

Turning the music up really loud, it drowns out all
other sound so it is much easier for you to tolerate.
Patient neighbours will be necessary for this one
though.

Craft activities

Completing an easy jigsaw puzzle.

Gentle cycle rides if you feel well enough are good as you are able to sit down. Can be easier than walking but must resist the temptation to do too much. Know your limits.

Going to the beach and walking in the water.

Spiritual activities e.g. going to church or meditating.

Cooking something nice for dinner.

Sewing/Knitting/Crochet

Cleaning the house.

Going to the hairdresser.

Visiting a spa/sauna.

Going for a manicure/pedicure or doing this yourself at home.

Photography

Building a model of something

Writing a letter to someone

Put up pictures on a board of things that you would like to do either now or when you get better. For example, holiday brochures, leaflets from somewhere you would like to visit; anything that makes you smile when you think about it.

Avoid puzzle books and reading things. Anything that may be mentally challenging will not be a good idea.

Often people will avoid going out on day trips to places as

they know they won't be able to do anything when they get there and it seems like a waste of money. Do it anyway. Just the experience of going out and seeing something will make you feel like you are doing things you would normally have done when you were well. Even going out and sitting in the car in front of a nice view can be good. Especially if you take a picnic and a pillow so you can fall asleep in the sunshine.

Although prior to M.E. a person may not have been very tactile this may have changed while they are ill. Patients often find that they are more emotional than prior to the condition, due to the brain's difficulty in regulating their emotions. As they are also likely to be more sensitive to touch they may feel more comfortable being hugged than they were previously. For those that do appreciate such contact it can also make them feel a lot better.

Permission Cards

There are many things that, as M.E. patients, we find ourselves getting stressed out about as we feel we should be able to do things when we actually can't. For this reason I am giving you some official get out of jail free cards. These are to be used whenever you like.

Official Permission to be Late as Often as you Like	Official Permission to Cancel as Many Unimportant Appointments as you Like
Official Permission to Wear Your Pyjamas All Day	Official Permission to not do any Housework and to not Feel Guilty About not Doing it.

| Official Permission to not be Sociable when you are out with Friends | Official Permission to do as Many

Things that you Enjoy as Possible. |
| --- | --- |
| | |

I often used to find it upsetting when people complained about how I had let them down yet again as I had had to cancel an appointment with them. Although they were aware that I had M.E. it was all too easy for people to lose their patience after I had had to cancel things on so many occasions. This is totally understandable, but very distressing if you are the one who cannot avoid doing this. The important thing is to not let this upset you. It is more important to cancel an appointment and rest when you need to, than worry about missing a coffee morning with a friend. Even missing a GP appointment is not going to cause a crisis, so don't push yourself beyond what you are able to do.

It is important to use the good days to prepare for the ones when you feel really unwell. Doing this will relieve your stress, as you know you have put things in place to cope with the bad days. Practical things, such as making dinners to put in the freezer so they can be microwaved later, can make a real difference. All of the things that you can put in place ready for the bad days will greatly reduce your stress for the days when you are really unwell.

But the main thing to remember from this chapter is......

Above all else, learn how to spoil yourself rotten!!!!!

4 SYMPTOMS

Symptoms and what can be done to treat them

This section will not contain a full list of symptoms but rather a few helpful hints on some of them. Please only read through the ones that are relevant to you. As the hypothalamus fluctuates throughout the course of M.E. we are all likely to experience different symptoms at different times so only some of these things are likely to apply to the individual.

Fatigue - Fatigue is often made worse by lack of attention to the other symptoms that are occurring. Your body is having to work harder to try to manage them and to compensate so you become tired out more quickly as a result.

Depression – Depression is not a normal part of M.E. despite the fact that a recommended treatment is to give the patient anti-depressants. The medicines contained in anti-depressants are actually hormones designed to make you feel good and the reason they are given is to rebalance the emotions so that the patient's symptoms are lessened. This is generally very effective so long as the right medication is given. There are many types of antidepressant out there so if you do not feel any benefit from one then I would recommend speaking to your doctor about trying a different medication. It is important to recognise however that some M.E. patients do end up genuinely suffering with depression due to the circumstances surrounding their condition. It is very important that they seek treatment for this as soon as possible. This is a completely understandable reaction given the life-limiting nature of M.E. Many patients who experience this may think that anti-depressants have no effect on the condition simply because they are on too low a dosage for their needs.

Anxiety/Panic Attacks – Anxiety and panic attacks during M.E. are usually caused by over-stimulation of the brain. This often happens in crowded environments with a lot of noise. Misconceptions of this problem may lead people to think that the patient is simply shy as they do not seem to cope well in social environments when it is actually their condition that makes it hard for them to cope. Such situations should be avoided if at all possible

28

and if unavoidable the patient should make sure that they regularly give themselves the opportunity to leave the room for a few minutes to prevent the build-up of anxiety. Anxiety and panic attacks can also occur at other times. As the brain is unable to manage the levels of hormones it produces it is not uncommon for it to introduce hormones into the body at inappropriate times. In this case adrenaline may be produced at random, causing the patient to feel very panicked and nervous. In this situation, try to eat or drink something sweet and go somewhere where you feel safe. A small room is good as you can become very aware of your surroundings, giving you a better understanding that the feelings you are experiencing are not real. This will fade quite quickly once you feel safe, but if it does not, seek medical attention.

Unusual Sleeping Patterns – Many patients become extremely worried about this, as this can often disrupt their daily patterns and steps are sometimes necessary to make sure that they are able to get back to a good sleeping pattern. It is not uncommon therefore for people to try to remain awake when their body is crying out for sleep and to try to force themselves to sleep when there body is telling them that it just doesn't want to. Medication can be used to work around this when it becomes extremely distressing for the patient but generally speaking the best way to stop this from happening is to just go with the flow. In other words, if you feel like being up at 2am and doing a jigsaw puzzle then do it; if you want to be asleep at 4pm in the afternoon, then why not? Sleeping at odd hours will not do you any harm and your body is more likely to get back to a healthy sleeping pattern more quickly if you don't argue with it and you do what it tells you to do for a while.

Feeling too Hot/Cold – It is important that you try to maintain a comfortable temperature for your body, regardless of what the weather is doing outside. If you are constantly feeling cold, then this lowers your immune system and makes you more susceptible to things such as colds and flu. Picking up illnesses such as this can be a major setback to your recovery, so at all times try to make yourself feel warm even if it means using a hot water bottle in July. Ice packs wrapped in a towel can be put in the bed if you suffer from being too hot or in reverse an electric blanket can be of real benefit. Feeling uncomfortable can make you feel very stressed, so for this reason it is also important to maintain control of this symptom.

Muscle Weakness/Blackouts – This can lead to muscle twitching or sometimes collapsing at random. I always found that I knew when my legs were about to give way underneath me and I developed methods for controlling this. Sometimes tensing all of the muscles in your legs can be enough to stop you falling at that moment. This is an effective way of controlling yourself until you are able to move to a safe place to sit down. Getting up too quickly can be enough to cause a blackout as your blood pressure suddenly changes so this should be avoided if at all possible. Standing still in the same place for any length of time will also cause the same problem, so sometimes gentle walking may be best when you are unable to sit down. In both cases of either muscle weakness or blackouts, patients can often find themselves collapsing at random. If you experience this then it is important that you learn how to fall correctly to make sure that you do not injure yourself. When you begin to collapse do not try to prevent it. Slightly tense the muscles down the length of your body so you can control yourself as you go down. Never fall sideways. Always let yourself go straight down by letting your legs give way underneath you. Once nearly on the floor allow yourself to fall on to your side. This takes practice but once learnt, can prevent injury from occurring.

Painful/Heavy Periods – Painful and heavy periods are very common in women with M.E. and most report a worsening of their symptoms around the time of their period. Hormonal changes take place in the body at this time which will again have an effect on the functioning of the hypothalamus. For this reason I would strongly recommend speaking to your GP about taking the contraceptive pill. Although this also uses hormones, it does provide a regular amount of such hormones and the regularity of this may be supportive. Blood loss can also be significantly reduced by the use of such medication so generally speaking the positives out way the negatives in choosing to do so. As always, discuss this with your GP thoroughly to make sure that this is an appropriate form of medication for you as an individual.

Sensitive to Light – Sometimes patients can have sensitivity to light without even realising it. This can often be subtle so trying a pair of sunglasses regularly for a while may be an idea to see if you feel better with or without them. Certain types of lighting can also be a problem, for example, shopping in a supermarket or attending school can become a challenge as the type of lighting in there can provoke mental confusion. Standard light bulbs are the best form of lighting for M.E. patients as these rarely cause any problems.

Sensitive to Sound/Smell – This is another symptom that can provoke mental confusion without the patient realising that the environment they are in may be the cause of this. Loud sounds are not a problem, but lots of little ones are. In M.E. patients, the brain has lost its usual ability to filter out sounds that it doesn't need to be aware of. For this reason the patient will be extremely aware of everything including simple things like a clock ticking, a tap dripping, a small pet playing in its cage. As the brain is unable to filter these things when a lot of little noises are present in a room the brain finds itself unable to cope and mental confusion occurs. It has to work extra hard to try to compensate for these things and therefore becomes tired more easily than if the noises were not present. The same situation occurs for patients who are sensitive to smell. The brain is unable to filter out what it needs to be aware of and what it doesn't so in this case providing things such as unscented soaps and bathing products may be extremely useful.

Sensitive to Touch – To explain this to someone who doesn't have M.E., the best way is probably as follows. You know that feeling when you have been sat on your foot for ages and it has gone completely numb, then all of a sudden the blood flow returns and the intense feeling that accompanies it is almost unbearable. Well that is what M.E. sensitivity to touch is like…..except it feels like that all over your body. Thankfully it isn't always quite that bad, but it is the same kind of feeling. Massage is the best cure for this. Not deep tissue massage, as this is extremely unhelpful for this and will probably make things worse. When I say massage I mean gently rubbing a hand lightly across the skin of the affected area. This can greatly relieve the symptoms, but make sure you avoid applying too much pressure as this makes the sensitivity worse rather than better.

Indigestion/Bowel Dysfunction – Please refer to the chapter on nutrition for advice. By having regular small meals, rather than larger ones, it is likely to improve these symptoms as the digestive system only has to cope with small amounts of food at any one time. If this is an ongoing problem however, speak to your GP who may be able to support you further. Indigestion can be greatly relieved by over the counter medicines designed for this purpose.

Bladder Dysfunction – Steroid injections can be really useful for this symptom. Once recovered however, the muscle weakness will not automatically return to normal. It is important therefore that if you have experienced any problems with this that you complete pelvic floor exercises until this returns to normal. Speak to your GP about this for further advice.

Mental Confusion – Mental confusion occurs whenever the brain has become overstimulated. It is very important to be aware of how this particular symptom affects you personally, as it is not only a hindrance to daily activities, but in some cases can lead you to put yourself in dangerous situations. If this is the case then try to make sure that you are not on your own whenever possible. The following things are likely to cause overstimulation; lighting, lots of little noises, being in a crowded environment, anything requiring concentration such as reading. Try to limit such activities as much as possible as this will greatly assist you towards recovery.

Extreme Hunger – Sometimes the body can produce excessive amount of the hormones that are designed to let you know that you feel hungry. This can lead you to the feeling that no matter how much you eat the hunger simply will not stop. It is not a pleasant experience and unfortunately there is not much that can be done about it. The important thing is to be aware that this is not genuine hunger and resist the urge to overeat. This symptom generally only occurs in the more severe stages of the condition but if it does, try not to worry about it. It will eventually fade. A warm, sweet drink such as hot chocolate can be really beneficial while this is occurring, the milk makes you feel as if you have eaten. It is important that this symptom is checked in case it is a sign of something unrelated to M.E.

Poor Vision – Poor vision can sometimes result from M.E. and this is usually linked to the fatigue. I would recommend regular eye tests and consider the use of glasses if required. I was concerned about doing this myself, but found that while I needed reading glasses when I had M.E., my eyesight returned completely to normal once I had got over the more severe stages of the condition. Using them at the time however allowed me to do things without feeling as tired.

For a full list of symptoms please refer to appendix 1.

<u>Working with your GP</u>

I would often go to see my GP when I was ill, but having spent all of my energy just trying to get there I was too exhausted to speak by the time I got into the room. Not very helpful! My GP would sit there and ask me what was wrong and all I could just about mumble was 'I don't feel well'. The GP probably thought I was a right idiot. 'Tell me something I don't know' I could hear him thinking to himself. The problem is that communicating with the GP for an M.E. patient is a far from easy process. Besides the obvious problem of being extremely exhausted by the time you get to speak to the GP there are several other factors here that often get in the way of good communication.

Firstly, the mental confusion that often accompanies being exhausted makes it hard to say what the problem actually is. This certainly doesn't help you when getting diagnosed in the first place and it is not much more helpful once you have. Even if it wasn't for this, the unfortunate reality is that when you have spent so many times going back and forth to the GP, many patients fear being labelled a hypochondriac.

But how does this affect communication? M.E. has a very broad range of symptoms but due to our fears about being labelled, we will often only mention one or two of the worst ones that we just can't cope with anymore. This however, is extremely unhelpful for the GP.

Generally speaking, the more symptoms a patient has, the more severe their condition. This is not always the case but it does tend to apply for most people. If the GP knows exactly what you are experiencing this is a good indicator of the level of M.E. you are currently experiencing. A rough guide to this is as follows:

Mild M.E.   0 – 10 different symptoms in an average week.

Moderate M.E.   10 -20 different symptoms in an average week.

Severe M.E.   20+ symptoms on a regular basis.

Another important reason for the GP knowing all of your symptoms is that this can help them to work out what symptoms they are able to treat. Many symptoms can be treated with medication but some medications cannot be taken alongside others. Managing as many symptoms as possible may be the best way to eliminate a patient's distress but priority should be placed on the symptoms that the patient finds most distressing rather than what is easiest to treat. The overall aim in treating the patient must be to reduce as much distress as possible for them to make an effective recovery.

Appendix 1 gives you a full list of possible symptoms that M.E. patients tend to experience. I would recommend that this list is used by GP's as a diagnostic and monitoring tool to manage a patient's condition. The pattern of symptoms is likely to change over a period of time so progress can be effectively monitored by repeating this assessment every couple of months. Although the patient's symptoms may have changed, the number of symptoms being reduced is the key indicator that they are beginning to get better.

Many patients who feel reluctant to communicate to their GP are a lot more likely to be open an honest about what they are genuinely experiencing if they are given a sheet such as this where they can just tick the boxes.

5 RELAPSE

What is a Relapse?

To describe best what a relapse is we need to think of the
brain as a very sophisticated computer. In this computer,
when it knows that it is malfunctioning it shuts itself down
in an attempt to reprogram itself. Putting this into
translation it means that when we have done too much
either mentally or physically, the brain says to itself –
'enough….stop…..I'm not doing this anymore. This isn't
working so I am going to reprogram the entire system'.

So the body shuts itself down by making you feel so
unwell that you don't want to get up or do anything. What
you will probably notice is that during a relapse, your day
to day symptoms do not particularly get worse but the
exhaustion and flu-like malaise gets very severe in

comparison to normal. The symptoms are a sign of the malfunctioning so they may have become worse in the days prior to relapse but will not continue to get worse once you are in it.

In forcing you to stop, the brain is allowing itself a chance to reprogram. With M.E., as the body's normal functioning has been disrupted it needs complete rest to be able to do this. This is a bit like when you set a computer to defragment itself. For the non-technically minded this is when you set the computer to sort out all of its files and re-organise itself. When it hasn't done this for a long time it can take several hours but once it has finished the computer works a lot better as it is running more efficiently. The computer does this entirely by itself once you have set the program in motion and in just the same way, once a patient rests fully, the body will know how to heal itself.

Despite all appearances, relapses are actually vital opportunities to get better. Just like the computer, it takes it's time to sort itself out and put all of its files and programs back in order. The more opportunities it has to do this the better it is able to work efficiently. The problem with this is that if you interrupt the brain half way through its reprogramming it gets even more confused than it was before and actually makes things worse.

Activity Management and Why this Fails

Activity management programs are designed for you to work out what you are able to do on an average day, without making yourself any worse and then gradually building up on what you are able to do. It is certainly true that prior to this assistance, a lot of patients make themselves very ill by doing too much of what they are not able to do and regularly end up having relapses. Clearly this is not a good thing for anyone. But what happens to the body when activity management is used?

When not following activity management, patients tend to end up doing too much, having a relapse, feeling a lot better again afterwards, doing too much again then having yet another relapse. A predictable pattern! But in an activity management program you learn how to stabilize your energy levels by only doing the level of activity that you can regularly cope with, without making you feel ill, and then sticking to that level as much as you possibly can.

After experimenting for a while you will find that you can do a certain amount of activity without making yourself ill and so you have found your day to day activity level. Great! It is definitely a good idea to work that one out. But what happens then? You will go along for quite some time without having any major relapses. Generally speaking you feel ill all of the time but it is better than having a relapse. Then, without particularly doing anything to bring on a relapse you suddenly find yourself in the middle of one. Frustrated beyond belief as you don't know why this has happened you go along with this for a while and when starting to feel a little bit better you go back to your normal daily routine even though following the relapse you struggle to get back to this over several days.

The following graph shows the energy levels you have during a relapse both of these scenarios.

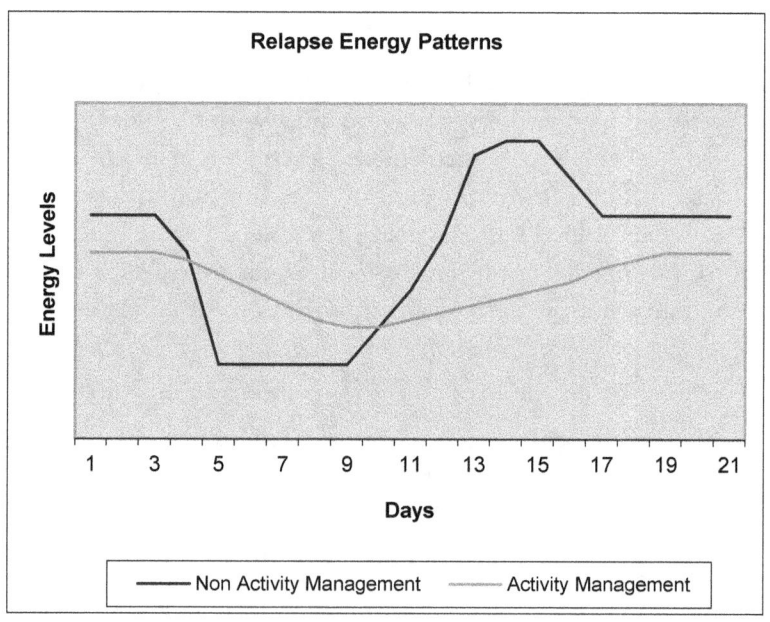

Now look at the difference. One very noticeable thing is that after having a relapse, when you are not following an activity management program, there is a period afterwards when you feel significantly better for a while. This doesn't happen when you are following the activity management program. But why is this the case? What is happening? And more importantly, how does this help us figure out how to get better?

In activity management programs the overall energy levels for the patient are on average lower than for those that do not follow them. The problem with not following them, is that although we feel better at some points, we also have times when we feel very ill.

The graph on the next page shows the pattern you need to achieve in order to get better. Although relapses still occur the period after them allows the patient to feel a little bit better than they did before. With this pattern, although there are still peaks and troughs, the general trend is towards increased energy levels over a period of time.

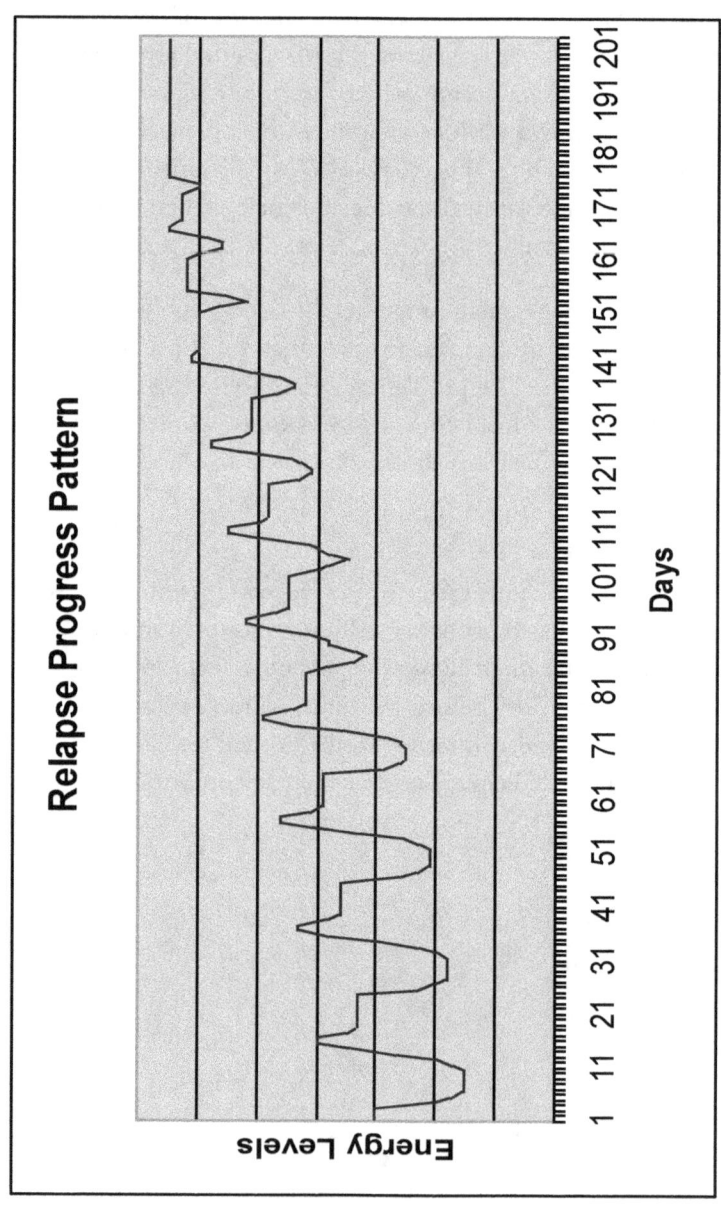

How to Manage Relapses Successfully

Two things are needed for you to be able to recover. Firstly, as mentioned before, you need to eliminate as much stress as possible. Secondly, you need to introduce a beneficial activity management program that allows you to make effective progress. The following are a list of rules that will enable you to manage your activity more effectively.

1. **Find out what you are able to do on an average day without making yourself feel ill.** This is exactly the same as standard activity management programs but with a key difference. **Only do this level of activity on an average day.** On the days when you are in relapse do not try to do this much. Sounds obvious, but this is a very important point as we will go back in a minute to define what exactly is a relapse day.

2. **As soon as you feel like you are about to have a relapse, stop what you are doing and go to bed.** Your body is telling you to rest and you need to listen to it.

Relapses have predictable patterns. You begin first of all getting some warning signs leading up to it. These are likely to be different for everyone so I can't tell you exactly what they are likely to be. Generally speaking your symptoms will start to get slightly worse than normal. In particular symptoms relating to mental confusion will probably be more noticeable than others. Learn to recognise these symptoms! The chances are that they will appear for a few days prior to the relapse happening. If you go to bed and rest at this point you can stop a relapse from happening. This does take practice but once you have learnt to recognise these things it can prevent a lot of problems for you.

The next stage is when you are in full relapse. You are both mentally and physically affected. Physically you don't want to do anything as you feel really ill and you will probably find that you don't want to exert yourself mentally either. By this I mean that you prefer to sleep rather than talk to someone or watch TV. Most people will allow themselves to rest fully at this point as their body will not let them do anything else.

The stage after this is the bit where people get tripped up. Mentally you feel well. You want to go out and do something. You want to sit up and watch TV. You feel like you should be able to do anything you want to as mentally you feel a lot better than you do on the majority of days when you have not experienced a relapse. The problem is that while you feel well mentally, your body is telling you something else. It just doesn't want to get up. The moment you try to get up you can feel your heart pounding in your chest. This of course seems understandable. You have just been through a relapse after all. So, despite the fact that we still feel really ill the majority of us start to reintroduce our normal daily activities. We are after all starting to feel better. Current advice says to work through this feeling so that the body is able to re-learn what is normal. WRONG. This is the worst thing to do.

When you reach this stage it is important to continue resting. What tends to happen is that people who have not had this advice will continue to rest. This is why people who have not had support will continue resting and feel much better afterwards while those who have been given activity management programs to follow take longer to recover.

It isn't easy to continue resting at this stage. Having to lay in bed for several days or even weeks is very distressing and it takes a brave person to do it. It is totally understandable therefore, that when we start to feel a bit better we get up and about whether we feel well or not. The important thing to remember is that if you can remain patient for a little while longer the benefits are innumerable.

3. **Do not get up until your body tells you to.** The trick with this is to monitor your pulse. This is absolutely the best way to make sure that you do not get out of bed before you are really ready to. When your pulse is still racing whenever you try to

get back to your normal routine – you are still experiencing relapse.

If you do not already know how to do this then ask your GP or nurse to show you how to measure your own pulse. This is really easy to do and is a vital skill in being able to get better. When you are not yet out of relapse, the moment you try to get up your pulse will go really, really fast. This is usually so noticeable when you have had a bad relapse that you can feel your heart pounding in your chest whether you try to measure your pulse or not. When you are resting in this stage however, your pulse will be quite slow.

Once you are actually ready to get up though this is completely different. Your pulse is then actually a lot slower than normal. Find out what your resting pulse rate is on a normal day when you are not having a relapse as this will make things a lot easier to work out later on. Use the graph on appendix 3 to record your pulse rate during a relapse. This will clearly show you your own individual pattern.

4. **Once you have got to the point where your body does really want to get up it is important that you do.** Once your body has reached the slower than average pulse rate stage you will probably feel like doing some mild exercise. Continue to monitor your pulse rate to make sure that you have really reached this stage. The best

thing to do is to try to go out for a short walk. While you are doing this you should notice your heart rate staying approximately the same. You should also notice a change to your breathing pattern. When in this stage you will find that when you go out for a walk the air feels really fresh in your lungs. Every step will feel like it is doing you a world of good even though you are not walking very far and are going really slowly. This will bring your pulse rate back up to your normal resting non-relapse rate.

By following these steps you should find that after the relapse you feel significantly better than normal. The trick is to remain patient. When in the more severe stages of M.E. just getting through the relapse can be one of the hardest things to do and it is important to ask friends and family to support you through this.

Having gone through the relapse fully you can then return to your average daily routine. Over time you are likely to find that the amount you can do on average will begin to improve. When the brain is allowed to use its relapses to reprogram itself properly it will start to make progress towards making you well.

5. **Above all, learn to listen to what your body is trying to tell you!**

6 FRIENDS AND FAMILY

Responding to others

Let's face it, we all have a relative somewhere that we don't like. A great aunt Mildred who will come round and sit there innocently sipping her tea, whilst peering over the top of her spectacles; her devious look makes you instantly suspicious, and without having any evidence at all, you just know that she has probably poisoned the Victoria sponge!

Leaving evil relatives aside for one moment, most of us have lovely friends and family who prior to our illness we have had really positive relationships with. Some of us are lucky enough to continue having that same relationship even after we are diagnosed, but this isn't always the case.

Many will notice that the way their loved ones behave towards them has altered and there are several things that are likely to be causing this.

1.   Problems being diagnosed.

A lot of patients find that they do not easily get a diagnosis which means that they are left for a long period of time with distressing symptoms and not knowing what is happening to them. This is just as difficult for friends and family to watch as it is frightening for us to experience it.

Just as we go through a process of emotions in this situation, those closest to us will also experience a range of feelings. The important thing is to try to re-open communication once you are diagnosed so that everyone is able to fully understand what is going on.

2.   Not feeling able to help.

Sometimes when people know that a loved one is in distress and they feel unable to help, they tend to convince themselves that they must be faking it. This is easier to accept than to acknowledge the fact that someone you are really close to is ill and you can't do anything about it.

3.   Not understanding what is wrong.

M.E. is a very confusing condition as it has so many different things that can be wrong at any one time. This makes it hard for other people to understand. A lot will assume they know all about it despite actually knowing very little which can lead to misunderstandings. If at all possible, encourage people to find out information about M.E. as well as talking openly with you about how the condition affects you.

In all of these cases people can tend to react negatively towards you but this does not mean that they don't care. It is important to remember that friends and family will be finding things difficult as well and their reactions towards you may be based on this. There are many things that can help in these situations to relieve the stress for everyone concerned and the following sections discuss these points.

When someone has been left undiagnosed for a long period of time it can be much harder to rebuild their personal relationships after finally being diagnosed. When such relationships have broken down as a result it may be best to stick to the facts when informing people of your diagnosis. Let people know what is wrong and then tell them how long it has been affecting you. This is unlikely to instantly change their opinions if these have been negative, but over time you may begin to see a change in their reactions towards you.

How friends and family can help

Having the support of friends and family can make a dramatic difference towards helping you recover. They can be a vital part of your support team, not only in physically supporting you but emotionally supporting you as well. If possible ask them to read this book so they have a good understanding of how to help.

The following is a list of things that friends and family can do to help if they feel able to do so.

- Giving you a hug.
- Doing the shopping.
- Bringing over a pet to visit if you are unable to look after one yourself.
- Loaning you DVD's to watch.
- Taking you out for a ride in the car or going somewhere nice.
- Taking you out on a picnic and allowing you to sleep while they do other things.
- Cleaning the house
- Making dinners to put in the freezer.
- Coming over to visit so you don't have to leave the house.
- Bringing over games to play or completing an activity with you.

- Being in the house even if you are just sleeping – it is nice to have company even when you can't do anything.
- Doing your hair/make-up.
- Giving you a manicure/pedicure.
- Giving you a massage.
- Putting some nice flowers in the garden or creating a window box for you to look at.
- Putting up a bird-feeder in the garden.
- Making a cup of tea/coffee.

The more support friends and family can provide the better; this will be of real value in helping the patient to get well as quickly as possible. Even the simplest of things take the patient a lot of energy to do so even making them a cup of tea will greatly help, as this is one less thing that they have to do.

Noticing the Signs

Friends and family can often notice the warning signs better than the patient can themselves. This can be really helpful for supporting them and the following are a few key indicators that you may find useful.

- Puffy eyes – When someone has M.E. it is very obvious as their eyes often look puffy. By this I mean that the soft area underneath their eye looks swollen and their eyes look as if they are slightly closed. This is a very good warning sign. In severe patients this is present all of the time, but for those who are less severe this comes and goes according to how well they are. If they have been quite well for some time and then you notice that their eyes start to loom like this then it may indicate that they are heading towards a relapse. If you point this out as soon as possible it may prevent a relapse from happening as they will know that they need to rest before things get worse.

- Slurred speech – An M.E. patient will often start to slur their speech in exactly the same way a healthy person would when they had drunk too much alcohol. This is easy for an outsider to overlook as they don't know that it is the result of their condition. This is a warning sign of being both physically and mentally exhausted, reminding them to go and rest is a good thing to make sure that they do not get any worse.

- Being emotional – This is a good indicator particularly in children. Frequent crying without being able to tell you why they are upset is a sign that they are both physically exhausted and mentally overwhelmed. Young children may also develop the tendency to hide when they feel like this as it makes them feel less vulnerable. As well as encouraging the patient to rest at this point it is important to support them by giving them a hug. Doing this will significantly reduce their stress and make a real difference towards helping them feel better. Talking will not make them feel any better as this is not a response based on real emotion.

- Confusion – When M.E. patients start to become overwhelmed mentally, you will notice it before they do. The mental confusion means that they can't see there is anything wrong with what they are doing. Besides the slurred speech you will also notice that they start making silly mistakes that they wouldn't normally make e.g. putting tea bags in the fridge, leaving an iron on, saying the wrong word when you know they mean something else. As soon as you notice this tell them. Make them aware of what is going on and tell them to go and sleep. This will quickly prevent the problem from becoming worse and can again prevent a relapse from occurring. This is also a key safety thing as it will prevent them from doing something that may be dangerous.

<u>What to do when you don't have people to support you</u>

A lack of support can make things a lot harder for someone with M.E. but there are many things that you can do to make sure that you are still able to make a full recovery.

To do this you need to create a good support network. The following factors need to be involved in this.

- A supportive GP/Specialist

- A group of people to talk to.

- Citizen's Advice Bureau/Social Services

- Practical Support

It is important to find a good GP/Specialist who you feel is both supporting and listening to you. Many people will stick with a GP they know simply because they have seen them for a long time. If you don't feel you are getting the best support for your needs however, it is important to see other people until you find someone that you feel comfortable with. Sometimes even personality differences can mean that you get on better with someone else. As this is someone that you need to have regular contact with it is important to get this right.

For those that do not have friends and family there to support them, it is vital that you find a way to access the internet on a regular basis. Support groups can often set you up with people to talk to who are going through the same things that you are. Having someone who understands is always a good thing and being able to chat via email or send letters can be a really good way to keep in touch with others. It is always better to see people in person if you can, so make every opportunity to do this where possible.

The Citizen's Advice Bureau can often help with important paperwork and Social Services may be able to provide you with a worker who can do things for you when you are unable to do them yourself. This can be of great support for sorting out your finances and other administrative tasks.

When qualified for Disability Living Allowance you should be provided with funds for your practical needs. You may find that you need to have a cleaner in once a week or to pay for shopping to be delivered rather than doing this yourself. Things such as dishwashers or tumble dryers can also be provided through this or even money for a taxi if you are no longer able to drive. Don't feel guilty about asking for these things. If you feel that this would really help you, then ask for it. Disabled badges for drivers can also be of real use.

One of the big problems for those without support is tackling the mental confusion. As this is not something that you always notice yourself, it can very quickly become a big problem before you realise that anything is wrong. Try to avoid any mental stimulation so that this problem is reduced. For good tips on how to do this please read the section in caring for severe patients as you can make similar adjustments throughout your home. As well as this it may be a good idea to put up several notices around your home. Make them brightly coloured so that you read them. Write on them the questions 'Am I struggling mentally? Am I starting to do strange things? If the answer is yes – go to bed'. These simple reminders may be all you need to stop yourself from experiencing significant problems. If you find you start to ignore the posters then re-write them on a different coloured sheet so that they regain your attention.

Support for Friends and Family

Joining in with activities that are there to de-stress the patient is a good way to not only support the patient, but to look after yourself as well. It is just as important that you spoil yourself as it is for the patient to do this. It is not easy to cope with watching someone live with M.E. and allowing stress to build up can only make this a lot harder than it should be.

Do not feel guilty about going out and having fun when you know someone is at home feeling unwell. The last thing they want is for you to suffer too.

If someone is feeling ill for long periods of time there are bound to be moments when they will get angry and say things that they don't mean. You know this person. Try to remember who they were before and know that what they would have said to you in this situation before they got ill is what they really would want to say to you now. They would tell you to go out and have fun. They would tell you to ignore them when they are being grumpy. Above all they would want to thank you for everything that you are doing for them at the moment. This person is still there. They haven't gone away. It is just that when you feel really ill all you can focus on is coping with your experience at that moment and nothing else.

It is ok to talk to the patient about how you are feeling. Don't try to hide it from them. They are still the same person you have always known and they will want to support you as much as you want to support them. Being able to support a friend when you can't do much makes you feel part of the real world again. They know that you are finding things hard and being able to talk to you about this can make them feel that they are able to give back some of the support that you are giving them.

Accessing support groups can be a good thing for you as well. Talking to other people who also have a loved one who is experiencing M.E. can be valuable support as they know exactly what you are going through.

7 NUTRITION

A Healthy Balanced Diet

Everywhere you look there is advice about eating a healthy balanced diet. 'Eat plenty of carbohydrate.' 'Don't forget your vitamins.' Another favourite at the moment seems to be that we are all supposed to eat five a day but the question is…..five of what? I suspect if I did nothing more than eat five peas off the end of my fork I would get some very strange looks from people if I proudly declared that I had had my five vegetables for that day.

So what does it actually mean? Roughly translated it means that we are meant to eat five different types of fruit or vegetables each day. The reason for this is that each different type of fruit or vegetable contains different nutrients so we need to eat a wide variety to make sure that we get all of the nutrients that we need. Simply remembering to eat a broad range of foods with plenty of vitamins and minerals as well as carbohydrate, dairy and protein should give you everything you need to make a full recovery.

A person's diet can sometimes be adjusted according to their current needs. For example, an athlete will need a diet with a lot more carbohydrate in it than an average person. But how does this apply to the average M.E. patient?

Surprisingly, the best thing you can do is to have a standard diet with an average balance of nutrients. The body needs all the vitamins and minerals to help itself to recover. It needs an average amount of carbohydrate to provide energy, but slow release carbohydrates will be better…or in other words eat brown bread and wholegrains rather than white. Protein is used to repair the body, so a slightly higher than average protein intake may be good but this won't necessarily make that much difference. It is more important to rest for the body to heal itself than it is to worry about dietary intake.

Eating when you don't want to

When it comes to M.E. the important question that I always had to ask myself was – how do you convince yourself to eat a healthy balanced diet when even lifting a spoon to your mouth makes you feel like you have run a marathon? Not an easy question to answer and one that I spent many years trying to figure out.

Trial and error eventually provided me with some answers but not, unfortunately, before I had ballooned to twice my normal size. This is what happened.

Convincing myself that there was absolutely nothing wrong with me I went off to Uni like every other 18 year old intent on having an extremely good time. Not so simple in my case you might think, and that prediction turned out to be correct. To try to cope with feeling exhausted all the time to the point I didn't even want to stand up I would drink glass after glass of coke. Not diet coke…the real thing. It worked though, for all of two seconds I felt a bit better…..can't say it was the cleverest idea though.

The coke drinking thing was not where it stopped. As I was too tired after coming in from half a day's study I couldn't manage to cook. Take aways were therefore the answer. Not even vaguely healthy ones. The only take away outlets on the student campus were the sort of thing that you could walk into and already feel the grease oozing into the pores of your skin. When I did manage to get some shopping, everything I cooked had to be done in five minutes or less. I could never manage to do anything more than that.

Needless to say this is not my idea of a healthy diet. If my Mum ever reads this part of the book I think she will pass out in horror at the thought of it and I will shortly be given a five hour lecture on the perils of take away food. The scary thing was, even at that age I did not want to be eating such an unhealthy diet. A lack of support left me feeling I had no other choice, and as a result, I did anything that would temporarily solve the problem. I doubt if I am alone in having been in this situation. Many M.E. patients who have limited support for whatever reason will either eat unhealthily or just won't eat at all. I eventually began to question how I could resolve this problem without having to rely on support from others.

Problem number 1

Looking at food that would normally be totally delicious but not wanting to even take a bite of it.

We all know the feeling of when you are just so exhausted that even if someone puts a gigantic chocolate cream cake in front of you, even the thought of taking a bite makes you feel exhausted. Not a good feeling. So what's the answer?

Bite size pieces.

If someone puts a great big thing in front of you it often looks too daunting to attempt. But if the same thing is broken down into lots of smaller pieces, it often becomes a lot more manageable and you also don't feel guilty for leaving any of it as it can be saved for later. This also works for trying to eat healthily. A whole apple looks intimidating when you don't feel well but the same size apple cut in to quarters is a lot easier to manage.

Problem number 2

Unhealthy food is loaded with calories and makes me feel better temporarily and also tastes better than most healthy food.

It is more important to make sure that you are eating something than to worry about how healthy it is. There are some days when you may feel that you are so tired that you either convince yourself to eat something unhealthy or not bother to eat at all. It is always better to eat something than not so don't be too hard on yourself if you don't end up eating the perfect healthy diet. Controlling your eating habits will be mentioned in the next section and this will help you too avoid the unhealthy cravings that come when we have pushed ourselves too far physically and are craving fatty/sugary substances to compensate.

Problem number three

I actually feel more tired when I eat healthy food than before I started eating.

It is easier to digest food that is soft rather than something that is hard. A lot of things that people consider to be really healthy such as raw foods like carrots & apples take more energy to chew and also more energy to digest. Soft foods are more quickly broken down so even during digestion soft foods take less energy to consume. As healthy foods also don't contain the high energy rush that you get from unhealthy foods this also makes them harder to eat.

Put into Practice

Eating a little and often is the best thing to do while you have M.E. This way you do not use a lot of energy eating or digesting food at any one time which is likely to make you feel exhausted. It has the added bonus of providing a steady amount of energy and nutrients throughout the day which is vital to making a full recovery.

Here are some sample dietary sheets for people with different stages of M.E. All of these are created in ways that should use low amounts of energy for you to create and to consume. Another tip I also learned is to make food in bulk and then store it in the freezer so you can reheat it later on. This takes a lot less energy to do when you are struggling to complete tasks.

Menu 1

Severe M.E. Patient

This menu should not be given at fixed points during the day but should be available to the patient at all times so they can snack on things whenever they feel able to.

Breakfast

1 Banana and yoghurt.

<u>Snacks need to be provided beside the bed at all times</u>

Nuts, Grapes, Cake cut into bite size pieces, mini sausage rolls, healthy crisps (e.g. Wholegrain), Sandwiches with healthy fillings that have been cut into eighths rather than larger sizes.

<u>Lunch</u>

Tinned Soup

<u>Dinner</u>

Casserole with all vegetables and meat cut into small pieces.

Menu 2

Moderate M.E. Patient

This should be a similar calorie intake as for a healthy person but is spread out across the day rather than in three set meals.

8.00am - Yoghurt with fruit cut into small pieces.

10.30am - A cup of tea with some biscuits

12.30pm - A sandwich cut into small pieces

2.00pm - A snack such as a sausage roll or some wholegrain crisps

4.00pm - Half a tin of soup

6.00pm - A small baked potato with a filling of the patients choosing and a glass of fruit juice.

8.00pm - A small bowl of healthy breakfast cereal.

Menu 3

Mild M.E. patient

A diet suitable for a patient experiencing mild M.E. may include harder food substances than more severe patients but should still be spread out across the day.

8.00am - Wholegrain toast with jam cut into small pieces.

10.30am - A yoghurt with some biscuits

12.30pm - A sandwich cut into small pieces and half a tin of soup.

3.30pm - A piece of soft fruit such as banana or kiwi.

6.00pm - Sausage casserole with mashed potato.

8.00pm - A small bowl of healthy breakfast cereal.

The following is a list of foods that may be good to use for M.E. patients

Soft bread (not crusty bread)

Bananas

Blueberries

Strawberries

Raspberries

Potatoes

Pasta

Fruit Juice (any kind)

Tinned Soup (really important as can contain a lot of different nutrients that are easy to digest)

Soft cheese

Milk

Any meat or fish

Tofu

Baked beans (make sure they are well cooked so they become very soft)

Yoghurt

Custard

Sponge Cake (not fruit cake)

Pizza made from wholegrain bread

Cereal

Porridge

Jelly

At all times it is important to remember that eating is a physical activity that does require energy for you to do. If you feel at any time that you are unable to eat then it may be that your body needs to rest a while longer before you can. If eating makes you feel generally worse during the day then you may need to adjust your eating habits further so it uses less energy.

8 BENEFITS, EDUCATION AND THE WORKPLACE

What benefits can you apply for?

Claiming disability benefits is not an easy process. There are so many rules and regulations that getting support is essential if you are to make a successful claim. If in the UK it is best to seek advice from both the Job Centre and the Citizen's Advice Bureau. They will be able to support you with making a claim and will be able to help you fill out the forms correctly. They can also provide you with the current information about what you are entitled to claim. This may change over time so it is important to keep in contact so you are aware of any upcoming changes.

Do not despair if you are not successful the first time you try to claim. Go back to your advisor and ask for further support as it may be that there is a simple reason that the claim was rejected.

At all times make sure you are completely honest about the level of support you need. There is so much help that can be provided, but if they are not aware of your needs then they can't arrange this for you. There are many things available that may be able to provide funds for mobility aids

How to support young people with their education

The information provided to schools on M.E. is still very limited so I would recommend that parents should try to have a meeting with the teachers to explain as far as possible what the condition involves.

A classroom environment is a very difficult place for a young person with M.E. to be in, let alone to try to learn anything while they are there. A classroom is filled with small noises that make it easy for them to become mentally overwhelmed. Chairs being moved, clocks ticking, people talking; all of it adds up to being over stimulated. Most schools have strip lighting in them which is also a nightmare for any M.E. patient.

School is the worst place for any young person with M.E. to try to make a recovery. If their condition is anything other than mild I would strongly recommend home tuition for a while until they feel better. As long as a child is being home-educated in some form then this meets the legal requirements, but it is best to work with the school to see if they can help you to set up something appropriate.

Homework should not be given as the young person is unlikely to be able to complete it. The teachers must make sure that their learning needs are met during school hours as they will not be able to do anything once at home. It does not help their emotional wellbeing if all hours are used up with study and they have no energy left to be with friends. Students may end up feeling like they have failed because they were unable to complete the homework tasks assigned to them.

It may be best for students to have an adapted timetable so that they are able to participate more fully. Most young people will study a broad range of subjects but for M.E. patients it is likely to be better to not continue with one or two subjects and to use this time as a rest period or time when they can complete homework tasks. This will need to be discussed with the school to work out what would be the most appropriate thing to do but generally making sure that the main subject areas are covered, such as English, Maths, Science and IT are good as well as any subjects that the student is particularly interested in. Getting fewer grades at a high level will look better to employers than a lot of mediocre ones.

In the school, teachers could be asked to change the lighting in the room to a standard light bulb which will make a real difference to the young person. This could be provided by a lampshade if it is not possible for the school to change the lights in the building.

The young person will not be able to learn when there is a lot of noise in the room so it may be an idea for them to sit in on the introduction to the lesson while it is explained what they need to do and then they could go to another quieter room to complete the task. It may be that one or two friends could accompany them to do this which would support them socially instead of feeling that they are being isolated.

It is very important that their peers understand what is happening and that they know what M.E. is. If the young person is happy for this to go ahead then it would be a good idea for a talk to be given to the class so they know why their fellow student has difficulty with certain things. When other children do not understand this it is very likely to lead to bullying and while it may be uncomfortable for the young person in the short term, the long term benefits of making their peers aware make it worthwhile.

Thinking about work

While choosing whether a child should stop attending school for a temporary period is relatively easy, it is a lot harder to make the decision about giving up work. Due to financial pressures people will often continue to work when they are really not able to and gradually see their health worsening over time.

Every person's circumstances will be unique to them so there is no simple answer about how to handle this. To prevent things from becoming difficult you will need to find out what all of your options are as soon as possible. Although you may not be feeling that unwell at present, preparing for the worst can relieve the stress we feel, simply because we have an action plan.

- Work out what benefits you can apply for and how much money you could claim.

- Find out if you will be able to continue living in your home if you have to claim benefits.

- If you will need to look for alternative accommodation, can support be provided from the council for you to do this e.g. Housing register for disabled people?

- If you choose to take time off and claim Statutory Sick Pay (SSP) then will this pay the bills and how long can you claim for?

- How long can you be off work for and still return to your job?

As always, the more stress you can relieve for yourself in this situation, the more likely it is that the worst case scenario won't happen.

The decision

The biggest decision that most patients and their families will face is when to withdraw from employment or education altogether. It isn't easy to decide this. Partly because it means acknowledging things really aren't that good for the patient as far as their health is concerned; but also because it is likely to have a big impact either now or in the future.

If a young person is still in the process of completing their education and they are finding this a real challenge then it is far better to take a break for a year and go back to it later than to struggle on. In that year they will make a lot of progress with their health if they have no other pressures to worry about. There will also be no gaps on their CV later that can't be explained, they will simply have taken their exams a year later or can record this as a gap year. A young person may want to stay in school for social reasons so it is important that they continue to attend a youth club or other social activities and they do not lose touch with their friends.

There are obviously going to be complications for any

person to give up work and this makes it extremely hard for anyone to decide what to do. The only advice I offer is to ask yourself a question; what would cause you the least amount of stress? If you feel so unwell that to continue to work makes you feel very stressed on a daily basis; is this more than you think you would feel on giving up work, then I say, give up work. If you feel that you would be less stressed in the long run to stay as you are, then do that.

Working part time instead of full time may also be a good option as this will allow you time to have the best of both worlds. I would strongly advise that you speak to someone about this before taking any action to make sure that you are fully prepared for all eventualities. If you are in a career that involves you being regularly stressed, then changing to something else temporarily may provide you with the break you need to get well again.

Remember above all, that once you are well again, things can be put back together. It may take a while to achieve this, but with the right support and motivation, it can be done.

9 CARING FOR SEVERE PATIENTS

Creating the Right Environment

Many severe patients are cared for at home by their families, while this is often because there is no alternative available, this can actually be the best environment for a patient to recover in. It is important, however, that the environment is set up to cater for the patient's needs. Although it may not be possible to make all of these adjustments, the more that can be made, the better able a patient will be to recover.

Light Sensitivity – It is important to have a thick pair of curtains at the window. Patients are likely to experience different levels of light tolerance at varying times and for these reason the ability to control the light is very important. Thin curtains will still let the light through but with thick curtains they can be part opened when required.

Sound Sensitivity – M.E. patients are often very intolerant to sound. When I say sound I do not necessarily mean loud sounds but often the lots of little sounds that are a part of our day to day experience. Remove any ticking clocks from the room. Stop dripping taps. Loud noises are not necessarily a problem but sudden ones are. Whenever possible the room should be kept as quiet as possible and ear plugs/muffs may be of great help.

Food – Providing regular small snacks for the patient may be a good way to avoid having to be tube fed. This also supports the patient's emotional wellbeing as they feel able to take some control over caring for themselves if they are able to eat independently whenever they feel able to. Please refer to Chapter 7 for further details.

Activity Management – It is important to remember that for severe M.E. patients the simplest of tasks are strenuous. Even something as simple as combing their hair or sitting up in bed can be an exhausting activity. If someone has reached this stage of the illness then the best thing to do is to leave them alone to rest as much as possible rather than to try to introduce any form of activity management. Encouraging them to do things that they clearly are uncomfortable doing is only going to prolong this stage further than necessary. The best thing to do is to allow them to do what they want to do and when they want to do it. It is more important at this stage to manage their mental well-being than anything else, but at the same time, monitoring their pulse rates will give a clear indication of what is going on.

Heat – Many M.E. patients have trouble controlling their body temperature so to ensure that they feel comfortable at all times, certain measures can be taken. For those who feel cold most of the time, an electric blanket can be of real benefit. If there are concerns however that this may be accidentally left on, then a hot water bottle would be better, but as this only warms one area of the body, things such as socks and gloves may also be of use. Wearing a dressing-gown in bed can also be extremely good as this is wrapped in tight to the body and will therefore make the patient feel warmer than just blankets alone. For patients who have a tendency to overheat the difficulty lies in being able to keep cool while not lowering the temperature in the house for everyone else. Although the obvious thing may be to remove the blankets and just have a sheet this can be unsettling as people often find that the absence of weight usually provided by blankets is missed. Ice packs usually put in food bags can be placed in the bed if well wrapped in a towel first. A fan or conditioning unit may also be helpful rather than leaving windows open.

Comfort – As the patient is likely to be more sensitive to touch, it is important to make sure that the bed they are lying in is as comfortable as possible. If the mattress isn't particularly soft then it may be an idea to put another duvet underneath the bed sheet as this will provide something soft to lie on without having to replace the mattress. Good bedding as well as plenty of pillows and cushions are always useful, but remember that when extremely exhausted the patient may prefer to lie completely flat without any cushions at all.

Hygiene – There may be some days when even being washed by someone else will be too much for the patient to cope with and may leave them feeling worse than before. The best thing in this situation is to leave them alone. It is better for them to rest and get better than to worry about washing. It is likely that within a day or two they will feel well enough to be able to do this then. Unless the patient is completely unable to do so, the best way to support them to wash is to give them a bowl of warm water and a cloth. Allowing them to do this for themselves not only allows privacy but gives them a sense of achievement that they have been able to do something. Hair washing should be left until the patient is able to have a shower as this is quite a tiring activity.

Supporting their Emotional Needs

One good thing about severe M.E. is that at its worst the patient's only wish is to rest as they are too exhausted even to think about doing anything else. This is actually a lot less distressing than when they are more awake and are able to notice their symptoms and what is going on around them. It is just as important to cater for the patient's emotional needs as it is to think about the practical ones. There is however a lot that can be done to support them during this time.

A patient may find it extremely hard to hear any sound in the room at all but that doesn't mean that visitors should be avoided. For those close to them it can make a world of difference to the patient if they are simply willing to sit there and give them a hug while the patient is allowed to fall asleep on them. This is the best medicine possible as the patient knows exactly how much you are supporting them. Other people may be able to sit in the room and hold their hand for a while. The feeling that they are able to continue resting while not feeling alone is extremely beneficial and will significantly reduce the stress that they are experiencing. There is nothing worse than going through this experience and being left completely on your own in the room constantly.

The best thing to do when you are completely bedridden is to develop a good imagination. When I experienced this myself I used my imagination to create a completely different life for myself in my mind. The important thing is to make this as exciting as possible so you don't get bored with it. As crazy as it sounds, imaginary friends can really be lifesavers. In my case I imagined being some kind of superhero, driving fast cars and causing all sorts of trouble.

I could never get bored of that one!

Support from family and friends and the use of your imagination are the two main sources of emotional support when in the severe stage. These are not to be underestimated as this is likely to be all that the patient either needs or wants during this stage. By making their environment as comfortable as possible and not encouraging them to do anything they don't want to is likely to be the most important form of distressing possible. All of these factors combined should help them to make steady progress.

Practical Support

Wherever possible it is important that the family get outside support if their loved one is in the severe stage of the condition. Unless you have a team of people around to support you then you are likely to wear yourself out to the point that you are no longer able to help in the way that you would like. A lot of support can be provided through the GP including practical support such as nursing staff if required. Cleaners could also be provided through money received from benefits which will free up your time for other things.

There are support groups out there for carers who can be

of invaluable assistance to those looking after all kinds of patients. I would highly recommend getting in touch with one of these, although you may feel fine with this for a while there will still be difficult days when having someone to talk to can be of real benefit. They can also provide a lot of advice on getting outside support and knowing which benefits can be claimed.

Looking after someone who is this unwell can be extremely stressful, it is important that you find a way to take a break and have some time for yourself, even if it is only for half an hour a day. A friend or relative could come over to watch the patient for a while so that you are able to go out yourself.

Unusual Symptoms

Severe M.E. can lead to some symptoms that are not generally seen in other patients. Here are a few tips for these that may be useful.

Mental Confusion

Patients can sometimes find that their mental confusion becomes so severe that they lose control of their understanding of what is going on. This is when they will start behaving like a child and humming to themselves.

This is actually not that distressing to experience for the patient as you feel like you are in a happy little world all of your own. If any friends and family recognize that a patient has got to this point it is very important that you encourage them to go to sleep so that the mind can rest. It is likely that they won't want to do this. They will likely recognize that they don't feel physically tired so will not want to sleep as they will identify sleeping with severe relapse. Going to sleep therefore is a frightening thought and the best way to help is to give them a hug and encourage them to sleep while being hugged. Once they do this the brain will begin to rest and they will then want to sleep as the brain switches into repair mode.

Breathing Difficulties

Unless someone has had a previous condition such as asthma then they are unlikely to have problems with their breathing, unless they are in the severe stage. Try not to worry about this. This is unlikely to become life-threatening; it is just very distressing to experience. Leaving this untreated however can be a big problem as being low on oxygen is not good for the body and makes it very hard to recover. For this reason, wherever possible, ask the medical profession to provide oxygen for the patient. If this can be provided it is likely to only be needed very temporarily. Breathing difficulties are more than likely to be caused by muscle weakness and therefore steroids may be considered as an option for treatment.

10 LIFE AFTER ILLNESS

Getting Back to Normal

For those that have only had M.E. for a relatively short
period of time it will be easy to get things back on track.
But for those who have had M.E. for many years it can be
a completely different story.

You suddenly find yourself landed in a completely new
world that, although familiar, is a strange land that you
barely even recognise. My advice is to take your time. Take
time to get to know yourself again. You will not be exactly
the same person you were before you had M.E., things will
be different; but that isn't necessarily a bad thing. It is not
always easy to do this when, for financial reasons, we have
to get back into employment as soon as possible.

Whenever possible though, try to reintroduce yourself to the world again slowly. After being limited in what you can do for so long, the prospect of being able to go out and do whatever you want can be extremely daunting. You find yourself going places that for so long were forbidden lands to which you dare not venture.

Take each day at a time. If you find yourself becoming overwhelmed, then the best thing to do is to stick to the routine you had while you were ill, but each day introduce a new activity that you were previously unable to do. A little and often can slowly help you return to normal.

Returning to your Career

M.E. for most will have disrupted either a person's career or education. Do not feel that because you have been out of things for a while that you have to settle for whatever you can get. Go to speak to a career's advisor in your local area. These are not just for teenagers but are for anyone who needs career advice. Take time to figure out what you would like to do and then write an action plan for how you are going to achieve it. It may mean re-training or possibly volunteering for a while. By volunteering you can gain current experience as well as a good reference that will be invaluable in getting employment. M.E. will have made a mark on your CV so it is best to gain advice as soon as possible.

Do not be afraid to speak to your former employers as they may be able to either give you a good reference or you may be able to apply for a position with them if there is one available.

Young People

If you have M.E. when you are young then you are likely to have missed out on some of the important experiences of growing up.

Some you may have had home tuition and may not have missed much of your education but others may have missed out on a large chunk of their studies. As with older patients, speak to a careers advisor about what to do next. You have plenty of time to retake your exams and do all the things you would like to do that will help you to achieve your goals. There are many different ways of getting back into education that are not commonly advertised by the schools.

Another important part of growing up is about forming relationships and discovering who you are and, unfortunately, there is a limited amount that you will discover if you are sat at home most of the time. As most people normally experience certain things at the same time as their peers it can be uncomfortable to have to learn this yourself later on. Do not try to rush to catch up on what you have missed. It is very tempting to do this but it will be a lot better for you in the long run if you take your time. All experiences will very soon be caught up on whether you try to make them happen or not.

PTSD and M.E.

M.E. is not a traumatic condition if you have been given the proper support and treatment. I am not saying it is easy because it certainly isn't; but for those who have experienced this for many years on their own it can often leave unseen scars that are left unspoken about.

When M.E. is not treated and recognized, the patient can go downhill quickly and can often end up in the severe stage of the condition. This is linked to not only severe stress but misunderstanding of the condition leaves us trying to push ourselves to do all we can regardless of what our body is telling us. It is easier to convince yourself that nothing is wrong than to admit that it is when no-one will help you.

For those who experience this and then later recover it can sometimes leave them experiencing Post-Traumatic Stress

Disorder (PTSD). A lack of support, regardless of how long you have experienced M.E., can also cause this condition.

Some of the symptoms of this are as follows:

- Difficulty sleeping
- Nightmares
- Hyper vigilance or easily startled
- Lack of self-worth
- Flashbacks or intrusive imagery
- Avoiding things that remind you of having M.E.
- Exaggerated startle response
- Keeping yourself busy and are reluctant to stop
- Putting yourself in dangerous situations
- Mood Swings
- Panic Attacks
- Addictions
- Being forgetful or confused

In particular, with M.E., you may find that you feel uncomfortable staying in the home as this reminds you of your illness. You may be reluctant to see your GP for anything, even when logically you know you should. Sleeping patterns may be a problem too, as you don't like the thought of having to be in bed.

Some of these things are a normal response to what you have experienced and are understandable under the circumstances. Most people will experience this in some form or another for a short time after recovery and developing PTSD is thankfully not that common. If these habits last for more than a few months however, and start to have a negative effect on your life, then it is important to talk to someone about this.

Support for PTSD can be given from your GP or a local independent counselor. Independent counselors can be expensive but there are some counseling agencies that can do things at reduced prices for those in difficult circumstances.

Relapses after recovery

You can sometimes find that although you have been fully recovered for quite some time you may occasionally find yourself having a mild relapse. You can usually do whatever you want to do, and then all of a sudden you will find that you start experiencing the familiar warning signs, a few days later you have a full relapse.

Do not panic about this. This does not mean that you have not recovered. It also does not mean that you are suddenly developing M.E. again. Despite having reached recovery the brain seems to take a temporary step back again as it begins to relearn what normal life is. I found that I could go for a year with no problems at all then suddenly would find myself having an odd random relapse.

These odd patches will eventually stop. It can take a few years after recovery for them to stop completely but even during this time you can go for a good six months or more without having any problems at all. Treat them as you would any other relapse and look after yourself for a while.

Muscle Weakness

If you have experienced M.E. for a long time and have also gone through some of the more severe stages of it then the chances are you will have developed muscle weakness. This is unfortunately not something that automatically disappears the moment you feel well again.

All of the areas of your body that you experienced weakness in while you were unwell, will need to take their time to rebuild themselves. Areas such as arms and legs will quickly regain their full strength as you use them regularly but other areas that aren't used as much may need to be worked on.

For example, if you had problems with bladder weakness then you may need to do some pelvic floor exercises to re-strengthen this. Even just trying to hold things a little longer before going to the toilet will help you to regain control.

It is a good idea to do a gentle exercise program on a regular basis for a while after recovery to regain your strength. Do not do anything strenuous. A little and often is the best approach. Swimming is particularly good for this as it tends to exercise most areas of the body.

The Secret

So here it is. The little secret that I cannot whisper to anyone, (except maybe in this book), it was the day I finally realised that I had completely recovered. Far from being a moment of anger and resentment it was the most exhilarating day of my life.

For weeks I had felt a lot better than normal. No major relapses; and I was starting to build my confidence with daily walks around the town. I had not felt particularly ill for some time but I thought that I was just going through a good patch and for that reason would continue with my daily routine as normal.

Up until that point I had continued with my daily life, normal tasks, nothing strenuous. The last thing I wanted to do when I was having a good patch was to bring on another relapse. Yet something in my mind began to question this. It was strange that I had gone for so long without feeling ill.

The summer came and each day I would walk out into the garden, feeling the warmth on my face. In sipping at the edge of my cup of tea the nagging thought would come daily into my mind. 'Go on, do it!'.

'Don't be ridiculous' I would always reply. "You'll only get ill again and then where would you be?"

Again and again this thought occurred. 'Do it' it said 'Do it...... do it!' After months of trying to push it to one side eventually I gave in.

At midafternoon I found the key to the garden shed. Looking towards the back I saw my rusty old bike that I hadn't been able to ride for years. 'Surely it can't do any harm if I go slowly and not too far.' After pumping the tyres and packing something to drink I gave it a go.

I had expected that by the time I had got as far as the bridge (less than a mile away) I would feel as lousy as anything. That familiar pang of 'Oh good grief, I shouldn't have done that' would come flooding through my body as if I had been shot with a poisoned arrow. Yet the bridge came and went and the air still refreshingly filled my lungs just as it always did after a relapse. I felt well. Better than that, it felt right.

On and on I went, not pushing myself too hard but not stopping either. I felt like a mad woman possessed. This was crazy. I'd completely fall apart the moment I got back. Yet that feeling of when you have over done it just didn't come. You know the one I mean. It's the one you try to ignore when you are having far too much fun. Yet it just wasn't there. Honestly it wasn't.

I got all the way along the road and back, twelve miles in total, yet I wasn't dead! I felt more alive than I had ever done in fifteen years! For fifteen years I had been a prisoner. Locked up for some crime that I never knew I had committed; and yet at that moment I was free! Free to begin my life over. Free from the pain, illness and suffering and yet more importantly free from M.E.

I will never be able to put into words how I felt that day. It was truly indescribable. The sunlight warmed my back and I looked at the world as if it had begun anew and given me a new chance to exist.

I have one thing left to say in this book and it is precisely this. M.E. is an horrendous experience. But in going through it for as long as I did it has given me a gift that can never be taken away. That feeling on the day I knew I had recovered has never left me. Each day begins anew and I can only be grateful that I am here to witness all the beauty in the world that it has to offer.

APPENDIX 1: SYMPTOMS LIST

M.E. Patient Symptoms List for General Practitioners

Please tick all of the symptoms that you are currently experiencing to help your GP support you fully. Please be aware that most patients are likely to only experience some of these symptoms at any one time.

Name ....

Date Completed ....

Anxiety/loss of confidence ☐

Blackouts ☐

Bladder dysfunction ☐

Bladder pain ☐

Bowel dysfunction ☐

Brain fog ☐

Breathing difficulties ☐

Changes in sexual appetite ☐

Confusion ☐

Constipation ☐

Depression ☐

Diarrhea ☐

Difficulty balancing/dropping things ☐

Difficulty sleeping ☐

Difficulty speaking ☐

Excessive sleeping ☐

Extreme feelings of hunger ☐

Feeling numb ☐

Feeling too cold ☐

Feeling too hot ☐

Fits ☐

Flu-like malaise ☐

Fatigue ☐

Hallucinations ☐

Headaches ☐

Indigestion ☐

Joint pain ☐

Memory loss ☐

Muscle pain ☐

Muscle twitching/spasms ☐

Muscle weakness ☐

Nausea/Vomiting ☐

Nightmares ☐

Painful/heavy periods ☐

Panic attacks ☐

Paralysis ☐

Pins and needles ☐

Poor vision ☐

Sensitive to light ☐

Sensitive to smell ☐

Sensitive to sound ☐

Sensitive to touch ☐

Sleeping in the day ☐

Sore throats ☐

Unable to stop thinking ☐

Vaginismus - painful sex ☐

APPENDIX 2: DAILY DIARY

With the mental confusion that often accompanies M.E. it is often easy to lose focus of what we want to achieve. Please feel free to use this diary to help you focus on the things that are important and also allow you to get better at the same time. It may be that just using this for a short while will help you to focus on what you need to do and enable you to get into a good pattern for managing your illness on a daily basis.

1. How stressed did you feel today? Give yourself a mark out of ten.

1   2   3   4   5   6   7   8   9   10

2. What things did you do today to make you feel less stressed?

a)...

b)...

c)...

3. How well did you do at managing to rest as much as your body wanted you to? Give yourself a mark out of ten.

1   2   3   4   5   6   7   8   9   10

4. How well did you do at sticking to a healthy diet?

1   2   3   4   5   6   7   8   9   10

APPENDIX 3: RELAPSE PULSE GRAPH

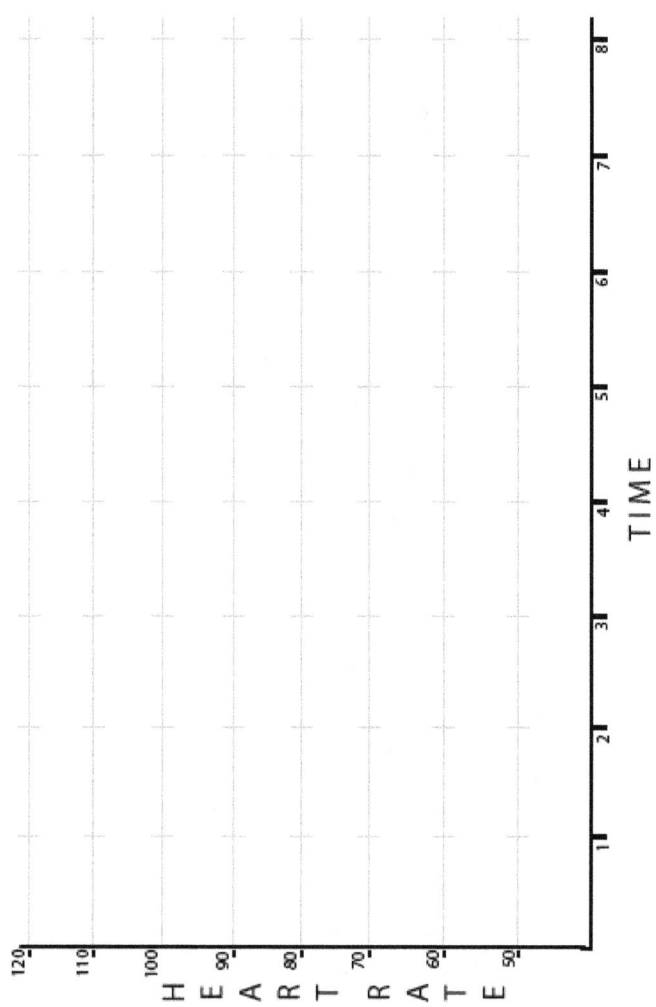

First Light of Dawn

ABOUT THE AUTHOR

L.S. Elmer experienced M.E. for 15 years. She had a gradual onset at first, but after a viral infection at the age of thirteen, she ended up in the severe stage of the condition for several years. After finally receiving a diagnosis after living with the illness for 10 years, she listened to all the advice given by the medical profession on how to get well. It didn't work. So being a bit of a rebel she began to question all of this and do things her own way. After an awful lot of trial and error, and doing exactly what she wasn't supposed to do, the answers slowly began to reveal themselves.

L.S. Elmer has now been fully recovered for 7 years. Despite being told this was impossible after having become as severely ill as she did, she has had no problems since and now leads a full active life as if she had never experienced M.E. at all.

www.ingramcontent.com/pod-product-compliance
Lightning Source LLC
Chambersburg PA
CBHW070538290526
45790CB00002B/544